20 MINUTES EXERCISE FOR PREGNANT WOMEN

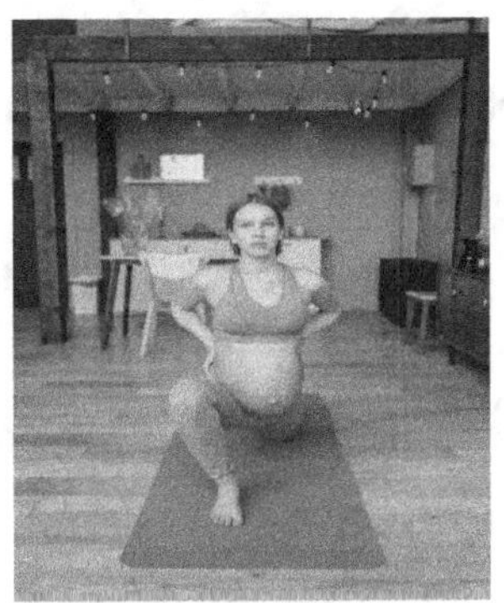

Elevate your well-being and embrace the benefits of tailored exercises for expecting moms.

By

Michelle T. Rills

Table of Contents

About the Book

Introduction

Foreword

Chapter 1

    1.1 Importance of Exercise During Pregnancy

    1.2 Safety Considerations

Chapter 2

Types of Exercises

    2.1 Aerobic Exercises

    2.2 Strength Training

    2.3 Flexibility Exercises

Chapter 3

Duration and Frequency

    3.1 Guidelines for 20-Minute Sessions

    3.2 Recommended Frequency per Week

Chapter 4

Exercise Modifications

    4.1Trimester-specific Adjustments

    4.2 Listening to Your Body

Chapter 5

Benefits of 20-Minute Exercise

    5.1 Improved Mood and Energy Levels

    5.2 Better Sleep Quality

    5.3 Reduced Pregnancy Discomfort

Chapter 6

Precautions and Contraindications

6.1 Medical Clearance
6.2 Warning Signs to Stop Exercise
Chapter 7
Sample 20-Minute Exercise Routines
7.1 First Trimester
7.2 Second Trimester
7.3 Third Trimester
Chapter 8
Post-Exercise Cooling Down
8.1 Importance of Cooling Down
8.2 Gentle Stretches
Chapter 9
Additional Tips
9.1 Hydration
9.2 Appropriate Clothing and Footwear
9.3 Monitoring Heart Rate
Conclusion
Quiz

About the Book

"20 Minutes Exercise For Pregnant Women" is a comprehensive and accessible resource tailored specifically for pregnant women seeking a balanced and manageable exercise routine. Authored by renowned prenatal fitness experts, this book delves into the importance of maintaining an active lifestyle during pregnancy while emphasizing a 20-minute daily exercise regimen.

The introduction lays the foundation by highlighting the benefits of exercise for both the physical and mental well-being of expectant mothers. Safety considerations take precedence, addressing concerns and precautions to ensure a secure workout environment for the mother and the developing baby.

The book categorizes exercises into aerobic, strength training, and flexibility routines, offering a diverse range of options suitable for various fitness levels. Clear modifications are outlined for each trimester, providing tailored guidance as the pregnancy progresses. This ensures that the exercises remain effective and safe throughout the different stages of pregnancy.

With a focus on practicality, the book provides sample 20-minute exercise routines for each trimester, empowering women to integrate these routines seamlessly into their daily lives. Post-exercise cooling down techniques and additional tips on hydration, appropriate clothing, and monitoring heart rate add depth to the guidance provided.

"20 Minutes Exercise For Pregnant Women" goes beyond a mere exercise manual, it serves as a holistic guide. With insights from healthcare professionals and a strong emphasis on individual well-being, this book becomes an indispensable companion for expectant mothers, promoting a healthy and active pregnancy journey.

Introduction

Embarking on the journey of motherhood is a transformative experience, marked by a tapestry of physical and emotional changes. Recognizing the profound impact of a healthy lifestyle during pregnancy, "20 Minutes Exercise For Pregnant Women" emerges as a beacon of guidance for women navigating the delicate balance of nurturing both themselves and their growing baby.

In this illuminating guide, we delve into the intrinsic connection between exercise and the well-being of expectant mothers, presenting a tailored approach for those seeking a manageable yet impactful daily exercise routine. The introduction serves as a compass, steering readers through the fundamental principles of prenatal fitness. It underlines the significance of maintaining an active lifestyle while fostering a deep understanding of safety considerations paramount to the unique dynamics of pregnancy.

Our commitment to empowering women unfolds through the categorization of exercises into aerobic, strength training, and flexibility routines, providing a rich tapestry of choices adaptable to diverse fitness levels. With a keen awareness of the evolving needs of a pregnant body, the book meticulously details trimester-specific adjustments, ensuring that every movement aligns harmoniously with the changing landscape of pregnancy.

More than a mere exercise manual, '20 Minutes Exercise For Pregnant Women' aspires to be a trusted confidante. Through sample 20-minute exercise routines, post-exercise cooling down techniques, and invaluable tips, we aim to equip expectant mothers with the tools to cultivate a holistic sense of well-being. This introduction sets the stage for an empowering exploration into the realms of prenatal fitness, laying the groundwork for a resilient and joyous pregnancy journey."

Foreword

In the quiet anticipation of motherhood, where every heartbeat resonates with the promise of a new life, '20 Minutes Exercise For Pregnant Women': A 20-Minute Exercise Guide for Expectant Mothers' unfolds as a narrative of strength, vitality, and the gentle rhythm of well-being.

Our story begins with a woman on the cusp of maternity, navigating the ebbs and flows of pregnancy with grace. In the opening chapters, we embark on a journey into the heart of prenatal fitness, where the pages echo the wisdom of experts and the heartbeat of a mother's intuition. It's a tale woven with the importance of cherishing one's body, understanding its needs, and embracing the symbiotic dance between the mother and her unborn child.

As the plot thickens, we delve into the diverse landscape of exercises, each chapter a new adventure offering choices that mirror the vast spectrum of a mother's strength. Aerobic landscapes beckon with the gentle rhythm of walking and the fluid embrace of swimming. Strength training unfolds as a hero's journey, with bodyweight exercises and light dumbbell workouts sculpting a narrative of resilience. Amidst the pages, prenatal yoga and stretching pose as poetic interludes, celebrating flexibility and the art of letting go.

The story arc gracefully navigates the trimesters, with characters named First Trimester, Second Trimester, and Third Trimester, each bringing its own challenges and triumphs. In this tale, safety is the protagonist, and modifications serve as plot twists, ensuring that every chapter resonates with the harmony of well-being.

And so, '20 Minutes Exercise For Pregnant Women' unfolds not just as a guide but as a companion, weaving a narrative that empowers expectant mothers to script their own stories of strength, endurance, and joy throughout the beautiful journey of pregnancy.

Chapter 1

1.1 Importance of Exercise During Pregnancy

Exercise during pregnancy holds profound significance for both the mother and the developing baby. Here are key reasons highlighting the importance:

1. Physical Well-being: Regular exercise helps maintain overall physical health by improving cardiovascular fitness, muscle strength, and flexibility. This contributes to better posture, reduced back pain, and enhanced endurance during labor and delivery.

2. Gestational Diabetes Management: Exercise plays a pivotal role in managing gestational diabetes by helping regulate blood sugar levels. It promotes insulin sensitivity, reducing the risk of complications for both mother and baby.

3. Weight Management: Proper exercise aids in managing weight gain during pregnancy.

This is crucial for the well-being of both the mother and the baby, as excessive weight gain can contribute to various health issues.

4. Mood Enhancement: Pregnancy often comes with hormonal changes that can affect mood. Exercise stimulates the release of endorphins, promoting a sense of well-being and helping to alleviate stress, anxiety, and depression.

5. Improved Sleep Quality: Regular physical activity is associated with better sleep quality. This is particularly valuable for pregnant women who may experience sleep disturbances due to hormonal changes and physical discomfort.

6. Preparation for Labor: Certain exercises, such as pelvic floor exercises and squats, can help prepare the body for labor and delivery. Strengthening these muscles contributes to better control during childbirth.

7. Reduced Swelling and Discomfort: Swelling and discomfort are common in pregnancy. Exercise, especially activities that promote

circulation like walking, can help reduce swelling and alleviate discomfort.

8. Enhanced Postpartum Recovery: Women who engage in regular exercise during pregnancy often experience faster postpartum recovery. Maintaining muscle strength and flexibility can aid in regaining pre-pregnancy fitness levels more efficiently.

Before beginning or altering an exercise programme, pregnant women should speak with their healthcare professionals to make sure it is appropriate for their unique health problems and the demands of their growing tummy.

1.2 Safety Considerations

It is crucial to make sure you are safe when exercising while pregnant. The following are crucial safety tips for new mothers:

1. Consultation with Healthcare Provider: Always consult with a healthcare provider before starting or continuing an exercise

routine during pregnancy. This is especially important for those with pre-existing medical conditions or complications.

2. Awareness of Body Changes: Recognize and adapt to the changes in your body. Modify exercises as needed, considering factors like balance, joint flexibility, and overall comfort.

3. Avoiding High-Risk Activities: Steer clear of activities with a high risk of falling, abdominal trauma, or injury. This includes contact sports, activities with a risk of falling, and exercises lying flat on the back after the first trimester.

4. Listening to Your Body: Pay attention to your body's signals. If an exercise causes pain, dizziness, shortness of breath, or discomfort, stop immediately and consult your healthcare provider.

5. Hydration: Stay well-hydrated, particularly during exercise. Dehydration can lead to overheating, which can be harmful during pregnancy.

6. Appropriate Clothing and Footwear: Wear comfortable clothing that allows for a wide range of motion. Supportive footwear is essential to maintain stability and reduce the risk of injuries.

7. Avoid Overheating: Overheating can be harmful to the developing baby. Exercise in a well-ventilated environment, stay hydrated, and avoid hot and humid conditions.

8. Pelvic Floor Exercises: Include pelvic floor exercises to strengthen these muscles, which play a crucial role in supporting the pelvic organs and can aid in labor and postpartum recovery.

9. Avoiding Supine Positions: After the first trimester, avoid exercises that require lying flat on the back for an extended period, as this can compress major blood vessels, potentially reducing blood flow to the baby.

10. Gradual Progression: If you were inactive before pregnancy, start with low-intensity

exercises and gradually increase intensity and duration over time. If you were active, you may need to modify your routine as your pregnancy progresses.

Remember, individual circumstances vary, so it's essential to customize your exercise routine based on your health, fitness level, and any guidance from your healthcare provider. Regular communication with your healthcare team ensures that your exercise plan aligns with the unique aspects of your pregnancy.

Chapter 2

Types of Exercises

2.1 Aerobic Exercises

Aerobic exercise during pregnancy offers numerous benefits, promoting both maternal and fetal well-being. Here's an overview of aerobic exercise considerations for expectant mothers:

1. Walking: Walking is a low-impact aerobic activity suitable for most pregnant women. It enhances cardiovascular fitness, helps control weight, and is easily adaptable to various fitness levels.

2. Swimming: Swimming and water aerobics are excellent choices during pregnancy. They provide a buoyant environment, reducing strain on joints while offering a full-body workout.

3. Prenatal Aerobics: Specifically designed prenatal aerobics classes cater to the unique needs of pregnant women. These classes

often incorporate low-impact movements, focusing on cardiovascular health and overall fitness.

4. Low-Impact Dance: Low-impact dance workouts, such as prenatal dance classes, offer a fun way to get the heart rate up without putting excessive stress on joints.

5. Stationary Cycling: Stationary cycling is a low-impact option that can be easily adjusted to suit individual fitness levels. It helps improve cardiovascular endurance without the risk of falling.

6. Elliptical Training: Elliptical machines provide a full-body workout while minimizing impact on the joints. Ensure proper posture and use the handles for stability.

When exercising aerobically while pregnant, keep the following safety precautions in mind:
1. Moderate Intensity: Aim for moderate-intensity exercise, where you can comfortably carry on a conversation. Avoid

pushing yourself to high intensity, and be mindful of any signs of fatigue.

2. Stay Hydrated: Drink plenty of water before, during, and after exercise to stay well-hydrated. Dehydration can affect both maternal and fetal well-being.

3. Proper Warm-Up and Cool Down: Begin each session with a gentle warm-up and conclude with a thorough cool down. This helps prepare the body for exercise and aids in preventing muscle soreness.

4. Listen to Your Body: Pay attention to how your body responds to exercise. If you experience pain, dizziness, or discomfort, stop the activity and consult your healthcare provider.

Before beginning or altering a fitness programme while pregnant, always check with your healthcare practitioner to be sure it is appropriate for your particular health circumstances and the demands of your growing baby.

2.2 Strength Training

Strength training during pregnancy can be beneficial for maintaining overall fitness and preparing the body for the physical demands of childbirth. Here's an overview of strength training considerations for expectant mothers:

1. Bodyweight Exercises: Exercises using your body weight, such as squats, lunges, and modified push-ups, are effective for building and maintaining strength. They help target major muscle groups without the need for additional equipment.

2. Light Dumbbell Workouts: Incorporating light dumbbells can add resistance to exercises, enhancing muscle engagement. Opt for weights that allow you to perform exercises with proper form without straining.

3. Resistance Band Workouts: Resistance bands provide a versatile and low-impact option for strength training during pregnancy. They offer resistance without putting excessive stress on joints.

4. Focus on Core Strength: Strengthening the core muscles, including the pelvic floor, can be particularly beneficial. However, avoid traditional abdominal exercises, especially in the later stages of pregnancy, and opt for exercises that engage the core without causing strain.

5. Proper Form: Maintaining proper form is crucial to prevent injuries. Focus on controlled movements and avoid rapid, jerky motions. Pay attention to posture and body alignment.

6. Breathing Techniques: Incorporate proper breathing techniques during strength training exercises. Exhale during the exertion phase and inhale during the relaxation phase. This helps maintain oxygen flow to both you and your baby.

7. Avoiding Supine Positions: After the first trimester, it's advisable to avoid exercises that require lying flat on the back for an extended period, as this can compress major blood vessels.

When engaging in strength training during pregnancy, consider the following safety tips:

1. Consult with Your Healthcare Provider: Always consult with your healthcare provider before starting or modifying a strength training routine during pregnancy. They can provide personalized guidance based on your health and pregnancy status.

2. Adapt to Your Fitness Level: Modify exercises based on your fitness level and any physical changes during pregnancy. Focus on what feels comfortable and safe for you.

3. Warm-Up and Cool Down: Begin with a warm-up to prepare your muscles and end with a cool down to promote flexibility and prevent stiffness.

Remember that individual circumstances vary, so it's crucial to customize your strength training routine based on your health, fitness level, and any guidance from your healthcare provider.

2.3 Flexibility Exercises

Flexibility exercises are crucial during pregnancy as they help maintain range of motion, reduce muscle tension, and alleviate discomfort. Here are some safe and effective flexibility exercises for expectant mothers:

1. Prenatal Yoga: Prenatal yoga is tailored to the needs of pregnant women, focusing on gentle stretches, relaxation, and breathing exercises. It promotes flexibility, balance, and a sense of calm.

2. Gentle Stretching Routine: Incorporate gentle stretches for major muscle groups. Pay attention to areas prone to tightness, such as the back, hips, and shoulders.

3. Pelvic Tilts: Pelvic tilts can help relieve lower back pain and strengthen the core muscles. Perform them while on your hands and knees, gently tilting your pelvis forward and backward.

4. Cat-Cow Stretch: This yoga-inspired stretch involves moving between arching your back (cow position) and rounding your back (cat position). It helps improve spine flexibility and alleviate back discomfort.

5. Seated Forward Bend: Sit with your legs extended in front of you and gently reach forward toward your toes. This stretch targets the hamstrings and lower back.

6. Butterfly Stretch: Sit with your back straight, bring the soles of your feet together, and allow your knees to drop to the sides. This stretch is beneficial for the inner thighs.

7. Side-Lying Leg Lifts: Lie on your side and lift one leg, keeping it straight. This stretch targets the outer thighs and hips.

8. Neck and Shoulder Rolls: Gently roll your neck and shoulders in circular motions to release tension. Be mindful of avoiding any sudden or jerky movements.

When incorporating flexibility exercises during pregnancy, keep the following safety tips in mind:

1. Warm-Up: Always begin with a gentle warm-up to prepare your muscles for stretching. This can include light aerobic activity or gentle movements to increase blood flow.

2. Avoid Overstretching: Aim for a gentle stretch without pushing yourself to the point of discomfort or pain. Pregnancy hormones can make joints more flexible, so it's essential to avoid overstretching.

3. Consistency: Engage in flexibility exercises regularly to experience their full benefits. Consistency is key to maintaining flexibility and preventing muscle stiffness.

As with any exercise routine during pregnancy, consult with your healthcare provider before starting or modifying flexibility exercises to ensure they align with your individual health conditions and the specific needs of your pregnancy.

Chapter 3

Duration and Frequency

3.1 Guidelines for 20-Minute Sessions

When engaging in 20-minute exercise sessions during pregnancy, consider the following guidelines to ensure a safe and effective workout:

1. Consult with Your Healthcare Provider: Before starting any exercise routine, especially during pregnancy, consult with your healthcare provider to ensure that the chosen activities align with your health status and pregnancy conditions.

2. Choose Safe and Low-Impact Activities: Opt for safe and low-impact aerobic exercises such as walking, swimming, or stationary cycling. These activities are gentle on the joints and provide cardiovascular benefits without excessive stress.

3. Incorporate Strength Training Exercises: Include strength training exercises using bodyweight or light dumbbells to maintain muscle tone and strength. Focus on major muscle groups and use proper form.

4. Integrate Flexibility Exercises: Allocate time for gentle stretching and flexibility exercises. This helps prevent stiffness, improves range of motion, and reduces the risk of muscle strain.

5. Warm-Up and Cool Down: Begin each session with a 5-10 minute warm-up to prepare your body for exercise. Include light aerobic activity and dynamic stretches. Conclude with a 5-10 minute cool down, incorporating static stretches to promote flexibility and relaxation.

6. Modify Intensity as Needed: Listen to your body and adjust the intensity based on how you feel. Aim for a moderate level of exertion where you can still carry on a conversation comfortably. Avoid pushing yourself to exhaustion.

7. Stay Hydrated: Drink water before, during, and after your workout to stay well-hydrated. Proper hydration is essential for overall well-being, especially during pregnancy.

8. Monitor Your Heart Rate: While there is no universal heart rate limit for pregnant women, use perceived exertion as a guide. If you can talk comfortably during exercise and don't feel overly fatigued, you are likely within a safe heart rate range.

9. Listen to Your Body: Pay attention to how your body responds to each exercise. If you experience pain, dizziness, or discomfort, stop and modify the activity. Always prioritize your safety and well-being.

10. Be Consistent: Aim for regular 20-minute sessions throughout the week to experience the cumulative benefits of exercise. Consistency is key in maintaining fitness and promoting a healthy pregnancy.

Remember that individual circumstances vary, so it's crucial to customize your exercise routine based on your health, fitness level, and any guidance from your healthcare provider. Adjust the guidelines as needed to suit your specific needs during pregnancy.

3.2   Recommended Frequency per Week

The recommended frequency of exercise during pregnancy can vary based on individual circumstances and health conditions. However, a general guideline is to aim for moderate-intensity exercise on most, if not all, days of the week. Here are some recommendations:

1. Cardiovascular Exercise (Aerobic): Engage in at least 150 minutes of moderate-intensity aerobic exercise per week. This can be broken down into sessions of 20-30 minutes, most days of the week. Examples include brisk walking, swimming, or stationary cycling.

2. Strength Training: Include strength training exercises for major muscle groups at least two times per week. These sessions can be incorporated into your overall routine, focusing on bodyweight exercises, light dumbbell workouts, or resistance band exercises.

3. Flexibility and Stretching: Incorporate flexibility exercises regularly to maintain range of motion and reduce muscle tension. Aim for 10-15 minutes of stretching after each exercise session or as a standalone routine.

4. Pelvic Floor Exercises: Perform pelvic floor exercises, such as Kegels, regularly. These exercises help strengthen the pelvic floor muscles, which can be beneficial during pregnancy and postpartum.

5. Rest and Recovery: Allow for rest days between exercise sessions to prevent overexertion. Listen to your body and modify your routine as needed, especially as your pregnancy progresses.

It's important to note that individual circumstances may warrant adjustments to these recommendations. Always consult with your healthcare provider to determine the most suitable exercise plan based on your health, any pregnancy complications, and your fitness level.

Remember that the goal is to maintain a well-rounded exercise routine that includes cardiovascular, strength, flexibility, and pelvic floor exercises. The emphasis is on staying active and healthy rather than pushing for high-intensity workouts. Regular communication with your healthcare team ensures that your exercise plan aligns with the unique aspects of your pregnancy.

Chapter 4

Exercise Modifications

4.1Trimester-specific Adjustments

Trimester-specific adjustments in your exercise routine are essential to accommodate the changing needs of your body throughout pregnancy. Here are guidelines for each trimester:

First Trimester:
1. Consultation: Inform your healthcare provider about your exercise plans and get their approval.

2. Maintain Pre-Pregnancy Routine: If you were active before pregnancy, you can generally continue with your pre-pregnancy exercise routine. However, be mindful of your body's responses and make adjustments as needed.

3. Focus on Core and Pelvic Floor: Begin incorporating exercises that strengthen the core and pelvic floor muscles. Avoid

exercises that involve lying flat on your back for an extended period.

4. Listen to Your Body: Pay attention to any signs of fatigue, dizziness, or discomfort. If you experience nausea or extreme fatigue, consider modifying the intensity and duration of your workouts.

Second Trimester:
1. Adapt to Growing Belly: Modify exercises to accommodate your growing belly. Avoid lying flat on your back and focus on exercises that maintain stability and balance.

2. Avoid High-Impact Activities: As your joints become more flexible due to hormonal changes, be cautious with high-impact activities to prevent injuries. Opt for low-impact options like swimming or stationary cycling.

3. Pelvic Floor Emphasis: Continue pelvic floor exercises and incorporate movements that promote posture and balance.

4. Stay Hydrated: With increased blood volume and the demand on your cardiovascular system, stay well-hydrated during exercise.

Third Trimester:
1. Further Adaptations: Continue modifying exercises as needed to accommodate your changing body. Choose exercises that reduce strain on the lower back.

2. Low-Impact Aerobics: Focus on low-impact aerobic activities to minimize stress on your joints and ligaments.

3. Pelvic Floor Preparation: Emphasize exercises that support pelvic floor health, including Kegels and movements that engage the pelvic muscles.

4. Listen to Your Body: Pay even closer attention to how your body responds. If you experience any pain, shortness of breath, or signs of overexertion, adjust or stop the activity.

5. Consider Prenatal Classes: Explore prenatal exercise classes tailored for the third trimester, which may offer specific guidance and support.

Remember, these are general guidelines, and individual circumstances may vary. Always consult with your healthcare provider to ensure that the adjustments align with your health and pregnancy status. Listen to your body, modify your routine accordingly, and prioritize safety and well-being throughout each trimester.

4.2 Listening to Your Body

Listening to your body is crucial during pregnancy, especially when it comes to exercise. Here's why it matters and how to tune in:

1. Sensitivity to Changes: Pregnancy brings about various physical changes. By paying attention to your body, you can be more attuned to these changes, such as shifts in balance, flexibility, and energy levels.

2. Individualized Approach: Every pregnancy is unique, and what feels comfortable for one person may not be suitable for another. Listening to your body allows you to tailor your exercise routine to your individual needs and comfort levels.

3. Warning Signs: Your body provides signals that can indicate whether an activity is appropriate. If you experience pain, dizziness, shortness of breath, or any discomfort during exercise, it's a signal to modify or stop the activity.

4. Fatigue and Energy Levels: Pregnancy often comes with fatigue. Listen to your body's cues regarding energy levels. If you're feeling tired, consider adjusting the intensity or duration of your workout or allowing yourself more rest days.

5. Adapting to Changes: As your body changes throughout pregnancy, your exercise routine may need adjustments. Adaptations may be necessary in terms of exercise type, intensity,

or specific movements to accommodate your growing belly and changing physiology.

6. Hydration and Nutrition: Pay attention to your hydration and nutritional needs. Pregnancy increases the demand for fluids and nutrients. If you feel thirsty or hungry, respond accordingly to maintain your well-being.

7. Emotional Well-being: Exercise can impact your mood and emotional well-being. If a particular activity brings you joy and relaxation, it's likely beneficial. Conversely, if something causes stress or discomfort, consider alternatives.

8. Consultation with Healthcare Provider: Regular communication with your healthcare provider is essential. If you have any concerns or questions about how your body is responding to exercise, seek professional advice.

Remember that pregnancy is a dynamic and evolving process. What feels right in one trimester may need adjustments in another. By listening to your body and making informed choices, you can create a safe and enjoyable exercise routine that contributes to your overall well-being during this transformative time. Always prioritize your health, and if in doubt, consult with your healthcare provider for personalized guidance.

Chapter 5

Benefits of 20-Minute Exercise

5.1 Improved Mood and Energy Levels

Engaging in regular exercise during pregnancy can contribute significantly to improved mood and energy levels. Here's how:

1. Endorphin Release: Exercise stimulates the release of endorphins, often referred to as "feel-good" hormones. These endorphins can act as natural mood enhancers, helping to alleviate stress, anxiety, and depression.

2. Increased Energy Production: While it may seem counterintuitive, expending energy through exercise can actually boost overall energy levels. Physical activity improves circulation and enhances oxygen delivery to tissues, promoting vitality.

3. Stress Reduction: Pregnancy can bring about increased stress and anxiety. Exercise

provides a healthy outlet for stress reduction by promoting relaxation and helping to clear the mind.

4. Better Sleep Quality: Regular physical activity is linked to improved sleep quality. The combination of reduced stress and increased physical tiredness from exercise can contribute to more restful nights, positively influencing overall energy levels.

5. Enhanced Self-esteem: Staying active can contribute to a positive self-image and a sense of accomplishment. This can be particularly valuable during pregnancy when the body undergoes significant changes.

6. Social Interaction: Participating in prenatal exercise classes or group activities provides an opportunity for social interaction. Connecting with other expectant mothers can offer support and contribute to a positive emotional state.

7. Alleviation of Pregnancy Discomfort: Exercise can help alleviate common

discomforts associated with pregnancy, such as back pain and swelling. Feeling physically more comfortable can positively impact mood and energy levels.

8. Cognitive Benefits: Physical activity has cognitive benefits, including improved focus and concentration. These benefits can contribute to a more positive mindset and increased overall energy.

It's important to note that individual responses to exercise can vary, and it's crucial to choose activities that align with your comfort level. Always consult with your healthcare provider before starting or modifying an exercise routine during pregnancy. Tailor your activities to your preferences, and listen to your body to ensure a positive and enjoyable experience that enhances your mood and energy throughout this transformative period.

5.2 Better Sleep Quality

Regular exercise during pregnancy can contribute to better sleep quality. Here's how incorporating physical activity into your routine can positively impact your sleep:

1. Stress Reduction: Exercise is known to be a stress-reliever. By engaging in physical activity, you can help manage stress and anxiety levels, making it easier to unwind and relax before bedtime.

2. Endorphin Release: Exercise stimulates the release of endorphins, the body's natural mood enhancers. This can create a positive and relaxed mental state, conducive to better sleep.

3. Improved Circulation: Regular physical activity improves blood circulation, delivering oxygen and nutrients to the body's tissues. This enhanced circulation can contribute to a sense of physical well-being and relaxation, promoting better sleep.

4. Regulation of Sleep Patterns: Consistent exercise can help regulate your sleep-wake cycle. By establishing a routine, your body becomes accustomed to a more predictable sleep pattern, potentially reducing insomnia and promoting more restful sleep.

5. Reduction of Discomfort: Pregnancy often brings physical discomfort. Exercise, especially activities that focus on flexibility and gentle stretching, can alleviate some of these discomforts, making it easier to find a comfortable sleeping position.

6. Energy Expenditure: Physical activity helps expend energy, making you feel more physically tired by the end of the day. This natural fatigue can contribute to falling asleep more easily and experiencing deeper, more rejuvenating sleep.

7. Temperature Regulation: Exercise can slightly raise your body temperature, and as your body cools down post-exercise, it may mimic the natural temperature drop that occurs as you prepare for sleep. This process

can signal to your body that it's time to wind down.

8. Consistent Timing: Try to schedule your exercise sessions at a consistent time each day. This routine can signal to your body when it's time to be active and when it's time to prepare for sleep.

It's important to note that individual responses to exercise vary, and it's essential to choose activities that are comfortable for you. Always consult with your healthcare provider before starting or modifying an exercise routine during pregnancy, and consider adjusting the timing of your workouts to avoid stimulating activity close to bedtime. Creating a bedtime routine that includes relaxation techniques, such as gentle stretching or deep breathing exercises, can further enhance the sleep-promoting effects of exercise.

5.3 Reduced Pregnancy Discomfort

Regular exercise during pregnancy can contribute significantly to reducing common discomforts associated with this transformative period. Here's how incorporating physical activity into your routine can help alleviate pregnancy discomfort:

1. Improved Posture: Strengthening core muscles through exercises like pelvic tilts and gentle abdominal work can promote better posture, reducing back pain and discomfort.

2. Enhanced Circulation: Regular physical activity improves blood circulation, reducing the likelihood of swelling in the extremities, a common discomfort during pregnancy.

3. Pelvic Floor Strength: Exercises targeting the pelvic floor muscles, including Kegels, can help reduce discomfort related to pelvic pressure and support overall pelvic health.

4. Reduced Back Pain: Strengthening the back and core muscles through exercises like squats, modified planks, and pelvic tilts can

alleviate lower back pain, a prevalent discomfort during pregnancy.

5. Alleviation of Leg Cramps: Regular calf stretches and ankle circles can help prevent and alleviate leg cramps, a discomfort often experienced, especially during the later stages of pregnancy.

6. Enhanced Digestion: Gentle exercises like walking can aid digestion and help prevent or alleviate common digestive discomforts such as bloating and constipation.

7. Management of Joint Pain: Low-impact activities like swimming and stationary cycling can help manage joint pain by providing a gentle form of exercise that doesn't put excessive strain on the joints.

8. Reduced Stress and Anxiety: Exercise is a natural stress reliever. By reducing stress and anxiety levels, regular physical activity can indirectly contribute to minimizing discomfort associated with heightened emotional states.

9. Improved Sleep Quality: Better sleep quality, often associated with regular exercise, can indirectly contribute to an overall sense of well-being and reduce feelings of discomfort.

10. Emotional Well-being: Physical activity releases endorphins, contributing to a positive mood. This emotional well-being can create a more positive outlook, mitigating the impact of various discomforts.

Always consult with your healthcare provider before starting or modifying an exercise routine during pregnancy, especially if you have any existing health conditions or concerns. Choose exercises that align with your fitness level and comfort, and listen to your body to ensure a safe and beneficial experience.

Chapter 6

Precautions and Contraindications

6.1 Medical Clearance

It's imperative to get your doctor's approval before beginning or altering a fitness programme while pregnant. This is the reason why:

1. Individual Health Assessment: Your healthcare provider can assess your individual health status, taking into account any pre-existing medical conditions, pregnancy complications, or other factors that may impact your ability to engage in certain types of exercise.

2. Personalized Guidance: Medical clearance allows your healthcare provider to provide personalized guidance based on your specific health needs. They can offer recommendations on the types, intensity, and duration of exercises that are safe and suitable for your unique circumstances.

3. Identification of Risk Factors: Your healthcare provider can identify any potential risk factors or contraindications to exercise during pregnancy. Certain conditions may necessitate modifications or restrictions in your exercise routine to ensure the safety of both you and your baby.

4. Monitoring Pregnancy Progress: Throughout your pregnancy, your healthcare provider can monitor changes and adjust their recommendations accordingly. As your body undergoes transformations, medical clearance ensures that your exercise routine remains aligned with your evolving health status.

5. Communication and Coordination: Establishing open communication with your healthcare provider fosters a collaborative approach to your overall prenatal care. It allows for coordination between your healthcare team and ensures that everyone is on the same page regarding your exercise plan.

Keep in mind that every pregnancy is different and that personal circumstances can change. You and your child may make educated decisions about the kinds and intensities of exercise that are both safe and healthy with the help of the information your healthcare professional provides. Exercise throughout pregnancy should always be your top priority. If you have any questions or concerns, speak with your healthcare professional.

6.2 Warning Signs to Stop Exercise

During pregnancy, it's crucial to pay attention to your body and be aware of warning signs that indicate you should stop exercising immediately. If you experience any of the following symptoms, cease your activity and seek medical advice:

1. Vaginal Bleeding: Any amount of vaginal bleeding during pregnancy is a red flag. Stop exercising and consult your healthcare provider promptly.

2. Severe Pain: Sharp or intense pain, especially in the abdomen or pelvic region, is a signal to

stop exercising. Pain should never be ignored or pushed through.

3. Dizziness or Lightheadedness: Feeling dizzy or lightheaded can indicate issues with blood pressure or circulation. Stop exercising, sit down, and seek medical attention if necessary.

4. Shortness of Breath Before Exertion: If you experience difficulty breathing even before engaging in strenuous activity, it's a warning sign. Consult your healthcare provider to rule out any respiratory or cardiovascular concerns.

5. Chest Pain or Palpitations: Chest pain or an irregular heartbeat requires immediate attention. Stop exercising, rest, and seek medical help.

6. Swelling, Pain, or Redness in the Legs: These symptoms may be indicative of deep vein thrombosis (DVT) or other circulatory issues. Cease activity and consult your healthcare provider.

7. Persistent Headache: A persistent or severe headache can be a sign of increased blood pressure. Stop exercising and contact your healthcare provider.

8. Reduced Fetal Movement: If you notice a significant reduction in fetal movement during or after exercise, stop exercising and contact your healthcare provider.

9. Amniotic Fluid Leakage: If you suspect your water has broken, which can present as a continuous trickle or sudden gush of fluid, stop exercising immediately and seek medical attention.

10. Contractions: Regular, painful contractions before the 37th week of pregnancy may be a sign of preterm labor. Stop exercising and contact your healthcare provider.

Always consult with your healthcare provider before starting or modifying an exercise routine during pregnancy. If you experience any of the warning signs mentioned above during exercise, prioritize your safety and seek immediate medical attention. Listening to your body and responding to warning signs promptly are key components of a safe and healthy exercise routine during pregnancy.

Chapter 7

Sample 20-Minute Exercise Routines

7.1 First Trimester

This is an example of a 20-minute pregnancy workout programme that is appropriate for the first trimester. Never forget to speak with your doctor before beginning a new fitness regimen, and modify the intensity to suit your comfort level:

Warm-Up (5 minutes):

1. March in Place (2 minutes): Begin with a gentle march to increase your heart rate gradually.

2. Arm Circles (1 minute): Stand with feet shoulder-width apart and perform forward and backward arm circles to warm up your upper body.

3. Side-to-Side Steps (2 minutes): Step from side to side to engage your hips and warm up your lower body.

Cardiovascular Exercise (7 minutes):

1. Brisk Walking (3 minutes): If you're outdoors, take a brisk walk. If indoors, use a treadmill or march in place with increased intensity.

2. Stationary Cycling (2 minutes): Cycle at a moderate pace. Adjust resistance as needed.

3. Low-Impact Aerobics (2 minutes): Engage in low-impact moves like gentle side taps or modified step aerobics.

Strength Training (5 minutes):

1. Bodyweight Squats (2 minutes): Stand with feet shoulder-width apart and perform squats to strengthen your lower body.

2. Wall Push-Ups (2 minutes): Stand arm's length from a wall and perform modified push-ups to target your upper body.

3. Seated Leg Lifts (1 minute): Sit on a sturdy chair and lift one leg at a time to work on your leg muscles.

Cool Down and Stretching (3 minutes):
1. Gentle Side Stretch (1 minute): Stand or sit and gently stretch your sides to alleviate tension.

2. Chest Opener (1 minute): Open your chest by clasping your hands behind your back and gently pulling your arms upward.

3. Calf Stretch (1 minute): Use a wall or sturdy surface to stretch your calves.

Pelvic Floor Exercises (2 minutes):
1. Kegels (2 minutes): Perform pelvic floor exercises by contracting and relaxing the muscles. Focus on proper breathing.

Remember to listen to your body and modify the routine as needed. If you experience any discomfort or if something doesn't feel right, stop and consult with your healthcare provider. Adjust the intensity based on your fitness level, and prioritize safety and well-being throughout your exercise routine.

7.2 Second Trimester

This is an example of a 20-minute pregnant workout that is appropriate for the second trimester. As usual, before beginning any new fitness regimen, speak with your healthcare professional and modify the intensity to your comfort level:

Warm-Up (5 minutes):
1. March in Place (2 minutes): Start with a gentle march to increase your heart rate gradually.

2. Arm Circles (1 minute): Stand with feet shoulder-width apart and perform forward and backward arm circles to warm up your upper body.

3. Side-to-Side Steps (2 minutes): Step from side to side to engage your hips and warm up your lower body.

Cardiovascular Exercise (7 minutes):
1. Brisk Walking (3 minutes): If you're outdoors, take a brisk walk. If indoors, use a

treadmill or march in place with increased intensity.

2. Stationary Cycling (2 minutes): Cycle at a moderate pace. Adjust resistance as needed.

3. Low-Impact Aerobics (2 minutes): Engage in low-impact moves like gentle side taps or modified step aerobics.

Strength Training (5 minutes):
1. Bodyweight Squats (2 minutes): Stand with feet shoulder-width apart and perform squats to strengthen your lower body.

2. Wall Push-Ups (2 minutes): Stand arm's length from a wall and perform modified push-ups to target your upper body.

3. Seated Leg Lifts (1 minute): Sit on a sturdy chair and lift one leg at a time to work on your leg muscles.

Cool Down and Stretching (3 minutes):

1. Gentle Side Stretch (1 minute): Stand or sit and gently stretch your sides to alleviate tension.

2. Chest Opener (1 minute): Open your chest by clasping your hands behind your back and gently pulling your arms upward.

3. Calf Stretch (1 minute): Use a wall or sturdy surface to stretch your calves.

Pelvic Floor Exercises (2 minutes):
1. Kegels (2 minutes): Perform pelvic floor exercises by contracting and relaxing the muscles. Focus on proper breathing.

Remember to listen to your body and modify the routine as needed. If you experience any discomfort or if something doesn't feel right, stop and consult with your healthcare provider. Adjust the intensity based on your fitness level, and prioritize safety and well-being throughout your exercise routine.

7.3 Third Trimester

Here's a sample 20-minute exercise routine suitable for the third trimester of pregnancy. As always, consult with your healthcare provider before starting any new exercise routine, and adjust the intensity according to your comfort level:

Warm-Up (5 minutes):
1. March in Place (2 minutes): Start with a gentle march to increase your heart rate gradually.

2. Arm Circles (1 minute): Stand with feet shoulder-width apart and perform forward and backward arm circles to warm up your upper body.

3. Side-to-Side Steps (2 minutes): Step from side to side to engage your hips and warm up your lower body.

Cardiovascular Exercise (7 minutes):

1. Brisk Walking (3 minutes): If you're outdoors, take a brisk walk. If indoors, use a treadmill or march in place with increased intensity.

2. Stationary Cycling (2 minutes): Cycle at a moderate pace. Adjust resistance as needed.

3. Low-Impact Aerobics (2 minutes): Engage in low-impact moves like gentle side taps or modified step aerobics.

Strength Training (5 minutes):
1. Bodyweight Squats (2 minutes): Stand with feet shoulder-width apart and perform squats to strengthen your lower body.

2. Wall Push-Ups (2 minutes): Stand arm's length from a wall and perform modified push-ups to target your upper body.

3. Seated Leg Lifts (1 minute): Sit on a sturdy chair and lift one leg at a time to work on your leg muscles.

Cool Down and Stretching (3 minutes):

1. Gentle Side Stretch (1 minute): Stand or sit and gently stretch your sides to alleviate tension.

2. Chest Opener (1 minute): Open your chest by clasping your hands behind your back and gently pulling your arms upward.

3. Calf Stretch (1 minute): Use a wall or sturdy surface to stretch your calves.

Pelvic Floor Exercises (2 minutes):
1. Kegels (2 minutes): Perform pelvic floor exercises by contracting and relaxing the muscles. Focus on proper breathing.

Remember to listen to your body and modify the routine as needed. If you experience any discomfort or if something doesn't feel right, stop and consult with your healthcare provider. Adjust the intensity based on your fitness level, and prioritize safety and well-being throughout your exercise routine, especially in the third trimester.

Chapter 8

Post-Exercise Cooling Down

8.1 Importance of Cooling Down

Cooling down is a crucial component of any exercise routine, and its importance extends to pregnancy as well. Here are key reasons why cooling down is essential:

1. Gradual Heart Rate Reduction: Cooling down helps gradually lower your heart rate. This gradual reduction is important to prevent sudden changes in cardiovascular activity, promoting a smooth transition from higher-intensity exercise to rest.

2. Blood Circulation Redistribution: After exercising, your blood vessels are dilated, and your blood flow is directed toward working muscles. Cooling down helps redirect blood flow more evenly throughout your body, preventing blood from pooling in

the extremities and aiding in the removal of metabolic waste products.

3. Prevention of Dizziness and Lightheadedness: An abrupt stop in exercise, especially high-intensity activities, can lead to a rapid drop in blood pressure, potentially causing dizziness or lightheadedness. Cooling down allows your cardiovascular system to gradually adjust, reducing the risk of post-exercise hypotension.

4. Minimization of Muscle Stiffness and Soreness: Cooling down includes gentle stretching, which can help minimize muscle stiffness and soreness. Stretching during the cool-down phase promotes flexibility, preventing muscles from tightening up after exercise.

5. Improved Flexibility: Incorporating static stretching during the cool-down enhances flexibility. This is particularly beneficial during pregnancy, as maintaining flexibility can help alleviate discomfort associated with changes in posture and weight distribution.

6. Enhanced Range of Motion: Cooling down with dynamic stretches can improve joint range of motion. This is important for maintaining mobility, especially considering the physical changes that occur during pregnancy.

7. Promotion of Relaxation and Mental Well-being: Cooling down provides a period of gradual relaxation, allowing your body and mind to transition from the heightened state of exercise to a more relaxed state. This can contribute to mental well-being and reduce stress.

8. Injury Prevention: Cooling down, including stretching, contributes to injury prevention by promoting balanced muscle development and reducing muscle imbalances that may lead to injuries.

For pregnant women, cooling down holds additional significance, as it contributes to overall well-being during this unique physiological period. Always listen to your body, and tailor your cooling down routine to your comfort level and individual needs during pregnancy.

8.2 Gentle Stretches

Gentle stretches are an excellent way to maintain flexibility, alleviate tension, and promote relaxation, especially during pregnancy. Here are some gentle stretches suitable for expectant mothers:

1. Neck and Shoulder Stretch:

- Sit or stand comfortably.
- Slowly tilt your head to one side, bringing your ear toward your shoulder.
- Hold for 15-30 seconds.
- Repeat on the other side.
- Avoid rolling your neck; keep movements gentle.

2. Cat-Cow Stretch (Modified for Pregnancy):

- Get on your hands and knees, with your wrists directly under your shoulders and knees under your hips.
- Inhale and arch your back (cow position), lifting your head and tailbone.

- Exhale and round your back (cat position), tucking your chin to your chest.
- Repeat for 1-2 minutes, moving slowly and gently.

3. Seated Forward Bend:
- Sit with your legs extended in front of you.
- Inhale, lengthen your spine, and exhale as you gently hinge at your hips to reach toward your toes.
- Hold for 15-30 seconds, feeling a stretch in your hamstrings and lower back.

4. Butterfly Stretch:
- Sit with your back straight and bring the soles of your feet together.
- Hold your feet with your hands and allow your knees to drop to the sides.
- Gently press your knees toward the floor for a stretch in the inner thighs.

5. Side-Lying Leg Lifts:
- Lie on your side, supporting your head with your arm.
- Lift one leg, keeping it straight, and hold for a few seconds.

- Lower it down and repeat on the other side.
- This stretch targets the outer thighs and hips.

6. Hip Flexor Stretch:
- Kneel on one knee, with the other foot in front, forming a 90-degree angle.
- Gently shift your weight forward, feeling a stretch in the hip flexor of the kneeling leg.
- Hold for 15-30 seconds and switch to the other leg.

7. Child's Pose (Modified):
- Start on your hands and knees.
- Sit back onto your heels while reaching your arms forward.
- Modify by spreading your knees wider to accommodate your belly.

8. Pelvic Tilts:
- Get on your hands and knees.
- Inhale and arch your back slightly, lifting your head and tailbone.
- Exhale and tilt your pelvis, rounding your back.
- Repeat for 1-2 minutes, moving gently with your breath.

9. Always listen to your body and avoid overstretching. Perform these stretches in a slow, controlled manner, and if you experience any discomfort or pain, stop immediately. If you have any concerns or specific health conditions, consult with your healthcare provider before engaging in any stretching routine during pregnancy.

Chapter 9

Additional Tips

9.1 Hydration

Hydration is crucial during pregnancy to support the well-being of both you and your growing baby. Here are key reasons why staying adequately hydrated is important, along with some guidelines:

Importance of Hydration during Pregnancy:
1. Blood Volume Expansion: Proper hydration helps maintain an adequate blood volume, supporting the increased demands on the circulatory system during pregnancy.

2. Nutrient Transport: Water is essential for transporting nutrients to the developing fetus. It plays a vital role in the absorption and distribution of essential nutrients.

3. Temperature Regulation: Hydration helps regulate body temperature, especially important as hormonal changes during

pregnancy can impact how your body handles heat.

4. Prevention of Dehydration: Dehydration can lead to complications such as urinary tract infections, constipation, and preterm labor. Staying hydrated helps prevent these issues.

5. Amniotic Fluid Production: Amniotic fluid, which surrounds and protects the baby, is mostly composed of water. Adequate hydration supports the production and maintenance of amniotic fluid.

6. Reduction of Swelling: Proper hydration can help reduce swelling, a common discomfort during pregnancy.

Hydration Guidelines for Pregnant Women:
1. Water Intake: Aim for at least 8-10 cups (64-80 ounces) of water per day. The actual amount needed can vary based on factors like activity level, climate, and individual health.

2. Monitor Urine Color: A pale yellow color indicates adequate hydration. Dark yellow or amber urine may suggest dehydration.

3. Spread Intake Throughout the Day: Sip water steadily throughout the day rather than consuming large amounts at once. This helps maintain consistent hydration levels.

4. Include Hydrating Foods: Incorporate hydrating foods with high water content, such as fruits (watermelon, oranges) and vegetables (cucumber, celery).

5. Listen to Thirst: Pay attention to your body's signals. Thirst is a natural indicator that your body needs fluids.

6. Avoid Excessive Caffeine: Limit caffeine intake as it can have a diuretic effect. Opt for water and caffeine-free beverages.

7. Hydrate during Exercise: If engaging in prenatal exercise, drink water before, during, and after to replace fluids lost through sweat.

Consult with Your Healthcare Provider: If you have specific health conditions or concerns, consult with your healthcare provider for personalized hydration recommendations.

9.2 Appropriate Clothing and Footwear

Choosing appropriate clothing and footwear during pregnancy can enhance comfort and safety, especially when engaging in physical activity. Here are some guidelines for selecting suitable clothing and footwear:

Clothing:
1. Comfortable Fabrics: Opt for breathable and stretchable fabrics like cotton and jersey. These materials provide comfort and accommodate your changing body shape.

2. Supportive Bras: Invest in supportive maternity bras to provide proper breast

support as your body undergoes changes. A well-fitted bra can help alleviate discomfort.

3. Loose and Layered Styles: Choose loose and layered clothing to accommodate your growing belly and regulate body temperature. Layering allows you to adjust for comfort in varying environments.

4. Elastic Waistbands: Look for maternity pants and skirts with elastic waistbands that sit comfortably below your belly. These provide flexibility and support.

5. Wrap Dresses and Tops: Wrap-style clothing is versatile and can be adjusted to fit your changing shape. It's a stylish and comfortable option for various occasions.

6. Maternity Activewear: If you're engaging in prenatal exercise, invest in maternity activewear designed to provide support and flexibility. Look for moisture-wicking fabrics to manage sweat.

7. Maxi Dresses and Skirts: Flowy maxi dresses and skirts are comfortable and stylish options that allow for movement and accommodate your growing belly.

Footwear:

1. Supportive Shoes: Choose supportive footwear with proper arch support. As your body undergoes changes, your feet may also experience some adjustments, so comfortable shoes are essential.

2. Low Heels or Flats: Opt for low heels or flats to maintain balance and stability. High heels can strain your back and may become uncomfortable as your pregnancy progresses.

3. Roomy and Breathable: Select shoes with a roomy toe box to accommodate potential swelling. Choose breathable materials to keep your feet comfortable.

4. Slip-On Styles: Slip-on shoes or those with adjustable closures (like straps or laces) are convenient as your ability to bend down may be limited in later stages of pregnancy.

5. Consider Arch Support Inserts: If your existing shoes lack proper arch support, consider using orthotic inserts to enhance comfort and reduce the risk of foot discomfort.

6. Anti-Slip Soles: Look for shoes with anti-slip soles to prevent slips and falls, especially if you're navigating different terrains during your daily activities.

7. Regular Foot Checks: Pregnancy can affect foot size, so periodically check that your shoes still fit comfortably. If needed, update your footwear to accommodate any changes.

Remember, comfort is key. Listen to your body, and choose clothing and footwear that provide the necessary support and flexibility throughout your pregnancy.

9.3 Monitoring Heart Rate

Monitoring your heart rate during pregnancy, especially when engaging in physical activity, is important for ensuring both your well-being and the well-being of your baby. Here are guidelines for monitoring heart rate during pregnancy:

Resting Heart Rate:
1. Normal Range: A normal resting heart rate during pregnancy is typically between 60 and 100 beats per minute (BPM). Individual variations apply, so it's essential to know your baseline.

2. Rest and Recovery: Pay attention to your resting heart rate in the morning before getting out of bed. An elevated resting heart rate might indicate the need for more rest or recovery.

Heart Rate During Exercise:
1. Target Heart Rate Zone: The American College of Obstetricians and Gynecologists (ACOG) generally recommends aiming for a target heart rate zone of about 60-70% of

your pre-pregnancy maximum heart rate during exercise.

2. Calculate Target Heart Rate:
- Step 1: Subtract your age from 220 to find your maximum heart rate (MHR).
- Step 2: Multiply your MHR by the desired percentage (e.g., 60-70%).

3. Modify Intensity: Pregnancy may affect your exercise tolerance, so listen to your body. If you feel comfortable and can maintain a conversation during exercise, it's likely safe.

4. Avoid Overexertion: Avoid activities that cause breathlessness, excessive fatigue, or make it challenging to talk. Overexertion can lead to overheating and potential risks for the baby.

Signs to Stop Exercise:
1. Dizziness or Lightheadedness: If you experience dizziness or lightheadedness, stop exercising and rest.

2. Shortness of Breath: If you're unable to carry on a conversation due to shortness of breath, ease up or stop.

3. Chest Pain or Discomfort: Stop exercising immediately if you experience chest pain or discomfort.

4. Excessive Fatigue: If you feel excessively tired or fatigued, give your body time to rest and recover.

Hydration and Body Temperature:
1. Stay Hydrated: Maintain proper hydration to help regulate body temperature. Dehydration can affect heart rate.

2. Avoid Overheating: Overheating during pregnancy can be harmful. Exercise in a cool environment, wear breathable clothing, and stay aware of your body temperature.

Individual Variations:
1. Consult with Healthcare Provider: Always consult with your healthcare provider before starting or modifying an exercise routine.

They can provide personalized recommendations based on your health status and any specific considerations.

Remember, individual variations exist, and what's suitable for one person may differ for another. Regular monitoring, staying within recommended guidelines, and paying attention to your body's signals contribute to a safe and beneficial exercise routine during pregnancy.

Conclusion

Incorporating a 20-minute exercise routine into the lives of pregnant women emerges as a holistic approach to promote physical and mental well-being throughout the various stages of pregnancy. The carefully crafted exercises, tailored for each trimester, serve as a practical guide to address the unique physiological changes experienced by expectant mothers.

The structured routines, encompassing cardiovascular, strength, and flexibility exercises, emphasize safety considerations and encourage regular physical activity, aligning with the consensus among healthcare professionals that exercise is generally beneficial during pregnancy. Moreover, the guidelines for 20-minute sessions, recommended frequency per week, and trimester-specific adjustments provide a flexible framework, acknowledging the dynamic nature of pregnancy.

Listening to one's body, a recurring theme in the guidelines, underscores the importance of individualized approaches. Each woman's pregnancy journey is distinct, and adapting the exercises to personal comfort levels ensures a positive and sustainable experience. The emphasis on safety considerations, medical clearance, and recognizing warning signs to stop exercise reinforces the responsibility of prioritizing maternal and fetal health.

The multifaceted benefits, ranging from improved mood and energy levels to enhanced sleep quality and reduced pregnancy discomfort, position these 20-minute exercise routines as valuable tools for fostering a healthy pregnancy experience. By integrating exercise into the daily routine, pregnant women can contribute to their overall well-being, potentially reducing the risk of complications and promoting a positive transition into motherhood. As with any health-related endeavor, consulting with healthcare providers remains essential to ensure a personalized and safe exercise journey during pregnancy.

Quiz

1. What is the recommended duration for a
    single exercise session during pregnancy?

A) 15 minutes

B) 20 minutes

C) 30 minutes

D) 45 minutes

2. During which trimester is it important to
    make specific adjustments to your exercise
    routine?

A) First trimester

B) Second trimester

C) Third trimester

D) All trimesters

3. Which type of exercise is generally
    recommended for pregnant women to
    improve cardiovascular health?

A) High-impact aerobics

B) Running

C) Low-impact aerobics

D) Weightlifting

4. What is a crucial factor to consider before starting any exercise routine during pregnancy?

A) The latest fitness trends
B) Consulting with a healthcare provider
C) Exercising only in the morning
D) Duration of previous workouts

5. Why is it important to monitor warning signs during exercise while pregnant?

A) To set new personal records
B) To avoid dehydration
C) To prevent overexertion and ensure safety
D) To compete with others

6. Which of the following is a key consideration when choosing appropriate footwear for exercise during pregnancy?

A) High heels
B) Low heels or flats
C) Tight shoes
D) No preference

7. What does the term "Kegels" refer to in the context of pregnancy exercise?

A) A type of dance move

B) Pelvic floor exercises
C) Breathing techniques
D) Abdominal stretches

8. How can you modify the intensity of your exercise routine if you experience shortness of breath during pregnancy?

A) Increase intensity
B) Continue at the same pace
C) Decrease intensity
D) Stop exercising immediately

9. Which trimester-specific adjustment is commonly recommended for pregnant women?

A) Increasing exercise intensity
B) Avoiding all abdominal exercises
C) Engaging in high-impact activities
D) Including more strength training

10. What role does monitoring resting heart rate play during pregnancy exercise?

A) It doesn't provide useful information
B) Indication of dehydration
C) Assessing exercise recovery and overall well-being

D) Evaluating baby's heart rate

11. Which type of stretching is generally
    recommended for cooling down during
    pregnancy?
A) Ballistic stretching
B) Dynamic stretching
C) Static stretching
D) PNF stretching

12. What does the ACOG recommend as the
    target heart rate zone during exercise for
    pregnant women?
A) 80-90% of maximum heart rate
B) 50-60% of maximum heart rate
C) 60-70% of pre-pregnancy maximum heart rate
D) No specific recommendation

13. What is a potential benefit of exercising
    during pregnancy for mood and energy
    levels?
A) Increased fatigue
B) Reduced mood improvement
C) Improved mood and increased energy
D) No impact on mood or energy

14. Why is it important to avoid overheating
during pregnancy exercise?

A) To prevent sweating
B) To avoid dehydration
C) Overheating has no impact
D) To prevent potential risks to the baby

15. What is a fundamental step before starting
any exercise routine during pregnancy?

A) Ignoring health concerns
B) Consulting with a healthcare provider
C) Imitating others in the gym
D) Starting with high-intensity workouts